I0415625

Table Of Contents

Introduction

Hot flashes, night sweats, irritability, insomnia, anxiety, and weight gain. Does this sound familiar to you? To the vast majority of American women, this and perhaps more symptoms, are the collection of an unwelcome and unpleasant experience they knew was coming: menopause.

If you are anything like my clients, you have likely tried many over the counter or perhaps even prescription recommendations before turning to natural medicine. And, if you are particularly new to natural medicine and don't know where to begin, the task of choosing a direction can be daunting. The amount of information on the Internet alone is endless with testimonials about this product and that herb. To make matters worse, conventional doctors are often unfamiliar with these products. So, they are unable to offer an opinion either way on whether you can stand to benefit from these possibilities or not. That leaves most women confused, frustrated, and without a solution to the symptoms of menopause they may be experiencing.

As a natural medicine practitioner, this is a picture I see quite often. And, happily, with a few simple recommendations, 95% of my menopause clients experience significant relief from their symptoms .... after only a few weeks of carrying them out. Relief from the constant irritability that threatens to ruin their

© 2013 Natural Health & Sports Massage Center, LLC. All rights reserved.

No part of this publication may be reproduced or transmitted in any form or by any means, mechanical or electronic, including photocopying and recording, or by any information storage and retrieval system, without permission in writing from the author (except by a reviewer, who may quote brief passages and/or show brief video clips in a review.)

Disclaimer: No portion of this material is intended to offer medical or personal advice. We've taken every effort to ensure we accurately and safely present these recommendations and their potential to help you. However, the information offered here is strictly for educational purposes only and is never intended to replace the individualized attention of a qualified health care/medical professional. Those with chronic illness or serious symptoms should always consult their doctor or other well-trained health care professional. Nothing in this presentation is a promise or guarantee of improvement in your symptoms. The content, case studies, and examples shared in this e-book do not in any way represent the "average" or "typical" client experience. In fact, as with any product or service, we know that some people purchase our material, never use it or don't follow appropriate guidelines, and therefore get no results from their efforts whatsoever. You should assume that you will obtain no results with the recommendations from this e-book. Therefore, the client case studies we are sharing can neither represent nor guarantee the current or future experience of other past, current or future clients. Rather, these client case studies represent what is possible with our recommendations. Each of these unique case studies, and any and all results reported in these case studies by individual clients, are the culmination of numerous variables, many of which we cannot control, including diet, lifestyle, sensitivity, follow up consistency, proper homeopathic case taking, remedy potency, remedy brand, and countless other tangible and intangible factors. Your level of success in attaining similar results is dependent upon a number of factors including your skill, knowledge, ability, and financial situation. Because these factors differ according to individuals, we cannot guarantee your ability to experience improvement in your symptoms. You alone are responsible for your actions and results in life and health, and by your use of these materials, you agree not to attempt to hold us liable for any of your decisions, actions or results, at any time, under any circumstance. The information contained herein cannot replace or substitute for the services of trained professionals in any field, including, but not limited to, medical, health care professional, homeopathic professional, or personal. Under no circumstances, including but not limited to negligence, will Cristina Villa Cantu, Natural Health & Sports Massage Center, LLC. or any of its representatives or contractors be liable for any special or consequential damages that result from the use of, or the inability to use, the materials, information, or improvement recommendations communicated through these materials, or any services following these materials, even if advised of the possibility of such damages. *Be advised that the client names, ages, and other identifying factors shared have been changed to comply with legal requirements and to protect the identity and privacy of our clients. In full agreement with the Texas Medical Board, Natural Health & Sports Massage Center is required to inform the public that naturopathic doctors are not licensed in Texas at this time. This means they are not able to serve as primary care physicians in Texas, however they can still be seen for consultation regarding health and wellness.

marriage, from the hot flashes that seem to strike suddenly and cause insufferable anxiety, and from the insomnia that causes a fatigue from which they can't seem to escape. Does that relief sound like something you would like to experience?

That's what this guide is about. When you finish reading this guide, you will know:

- What you have been doing that is likely making your menopause symptoms worse.
- What you need to start doing in order to create a solid foundation for healing.
- The secret weapon most women don't know about that can offer swift relief from the symptoms of menopause.

To make it easier to approach, this guide has been laid out in steps. There are four of them and they complement each other. They are simple, actionable, and **_effective_**. That last word there is bolded for a reason. The steps that I have laid out in this guide are the ones that I have seen work consistently for hundreds of menopause clients. Are there other natural therapies that might hold some promise? To be sure! But these are the most effective most consistently. And this is about showing you what works, not what might work.

I can list you pages of herbs and supplements that can all possibly help with different aspects of menopause. The problem with this approach for many women is that it doesn't take their particular picture into consideration. They might have hot flashes, but the supplement they choose doesn't address their bloating or fatigue. Or maybe they have anxiety, but the herb they choose doesn't address their migraines or their night sweats. This usually leads to a menopausal woman on multiple different products and unsure of which is doing what.

After seeing hundreds of clients with menopause, it has become quite obvious that every woman is different. Every experience of menopause is unique to the individual. Sure, they might share some mutual symptoms but it would be ludicrous to reduce their experience to a common medical diagnosis, slap them on whatever synthetic craze is popular at the moment, and expect phenomenal results without repercussions. While that approach might work for some, it has become increasingly evident that today's menopausal women are looking for more. A more personalized approach that addresses their whole picture and is safer, gentler, and actually works. That's what this guide is about.

The nice thing about this guide is that these steps can be used in any order at all. They don't have to be done in the order that is outlined. And even though the steps are meant to be done together and will have the most impact that way, they don't have to be. You can pick and choose as you wish. Often, we need encouragement or proof that natural medicine might "work" for us before we are ready to commit to it with dedication. And that is completely understandable. I have many clients that have tried step 1, saw incredible results, and then went on to adopt the rest of the steps. The reasoning is obvious: 'If I feel this good with just this step, how much better will I feel with more?'

Without much more, I encourage you to dive in and learn about the possibilities that can help transform your experience of menopause to a more positive one. You will see success stories from some of my very own clients sprinkled here and there about different steps they chose to focus on and what it has done for them. These are real life examples of how normal, everyday people incorporated these simple steps into their lives and saw profound results. I hope you enjoy hearing about their journey as much as I did. Here's to your health and the next, exciting chapter of your life.

-Cristina Villa Cantu
Natural Medicine Practitioner
www.justnaturalremedies.com

Step 1: Foods to Avoid

Discover What's Making You Feel Worse

The first two steps are devoted entirely to diet because food can be an incredibly effective tool at helping quell or flare the symptoms of menopause. When you finish reading these steps you will know:

- what foods to stay away from and why
- what foods to eat more of and how much of them

It will be easier to start with what foods to stay away from so that we get the "bad news" out of the way first. For some women, this step alone can be the **only one** they'll ever have to take in order to reduce their menopause symptoms. It is ***that*** powerful. Here are the major food culprits that aggravate common menopause symptoms and why they do so.

Caffeine

That cup of coffee may jump start your day, but it can also cause your blood sugar levels to drop rapidly. This blood sugar yo-yo can aggravate mood swings, depression and irritability, all of which are among the biggest concerns for menopausal women. This can make you hungry more often, causing you to eat more often and gain weight as a result. Weight gain is also something that many women going through menopause repot they struggle with.

Also, caffeine is a well-documented cause of insomnia, which menopausal women frequently express concern about. Not only because it won't let them fall asleep at night, but because it increases the amount of times they have to get up to go the bathroom at night. This seems to hold especially true if the caffeine is consumed later in the day.

As if that weren't enough, research shows women who drank two cups of coffee a day or more were more likely to experience hot flashes than women who didn't drink coffee at all.[1] For 90% of the women that I have seen, they report this is true. Hot flashes are the number one concern among all my menopause clients, so this piece of information is particularly important. The correlation between cups of coffee consumed and the incidence of hot flashes seems directly proportional, meaning the more coffee women drink, the more likely they are to experience hot flashes. Not only that, the intensity of their hot flashes seems to increase.

Finally, caffeine is a drying substance. Increased consumption of caffeine related products increases the likelihood of vaginal dryness, a common concern among menopausal women. This can lead to urinary problems such as urinary urgency or bladder infections, as well as painful intercourse.

---

[1] http://www.breastcancer.org/tips/menopausal/facing/hot_flashes

Future Concerns of Caffeine Consumption

Along with the symptoms that you may be experiencing now, caffeine can have an impact on important areas of your health that you need to be aware of to keep your health at its optimal level.

Caffeine is very good at leaching calcium out of your bones, increasing your risk of developing osteoporosis and bone fractures in the future. Not only that, since it causes you to urinate more often it may, over time, contribute to a vitamin and mineral deficiency. This would happen over a long period of time, not right away and is quite difficult to achieve. But with a poor diet and lifestyle, it's not implausible. As we age, it is harder to restore this balance than you would think, and can contribute to a wide variety of mental and physical conditions that are avoidable.

Sugar

Most people have an addiction, in some form or other, to refined sugar. If you maintain a standard American diet (also known as SAD…. ironic, don't you think?), chances are excellent that you consume sugar not only in the foods you eat, but also in the drinks you drink. The average American consumes 22 teaspoons of sugar per day (that's 10 times more than any other food additive), and most of that is attributed to soft drinks.[2] And when you consider sugar's strong link to obesity, diabetes, hypertension, depression, fatigue, headaches, and more, this

---

[2] http://www.forbes.com/sites/alicegwalton/2012/08/30/how-much-sugar-are-americans-eating-infographic/

number appears not only outrageous, but downright frightening. But let's consider its effect on the common menopausal woman.

When refined sugar is consumed without a ride along buddy like protein or fiber, which is often the rule and not the exception with most people, it spikes your blood sugar level to the point where your body needs to step in and handle the "problem". And handle the problem it does, at the expense of your mental/emotional well being causing your blood sugar levels to drop back down pretty rapidly. This is the blood sugar yo-yo we talked about when we discussed caffeine that has been shown to negatively impact hormone balance, making depression, mood swings, and irritability worse.

As we already mentioned, it's no secret and there are pounds of research that support refined sugar's irrefutable association with obesity. For about 73% of the menopausal women that I have seen, weight gain is a significant concern. For many of them, cutting refined sugar out of their diet alone helps them maintain a steady blood glucose level. This, they report, significantly contributes to a more balanced mental/emotional state, as well as curbs their cravings for sweet snacks, helping them avoid the foods that would have caused them to gain weight.

If refined sugar is consumed close to bedtime, you can look forward to the blood sugar yo-yo happening while you sleep. This can be responsible for causing insomnia and early morning headaches because blood sugar levels are too low. Many menopausal women report having trouble with falling or staying asleep, which makes steering clear of this practice a good idea.

Lastly, sugar makes it very easy for yeast to grow in your tissues. For women going through menopause, vaginal infections will be one of the top things to know about and prevent, as yeast can easily support a chronic vaginal infection. Avoiding a diet high in sugar can make this particular issue one less thing to worry about.

Future Concerns of Sugar Consumption
Refined sugar is very good at aggravating musculoskeletal concerns such as aches, pains, and rheumatism. Although it is not clear yet whether sugar actually causes arthritis and other related concerns, it is clear that people with these concerns experience relief from their symptoms when they omit sugar from their diet.

Additionally, cancer and sugar have been shown to have an interesting association. Although cancer is caused by a myriad of different factors, the research is clear about how cancer survives once it is around. Among other things it eats to live, sugar is its substance of choice. Why should this be important to you? Here's what we know:

- A diet high in sugar will depress your overall immune system, leaving you more vulnerable to common colds, flus, and infections (acute illness).
- If you do happen to fall acutely ill, you will stay sick longer if you maintain a high sugar diet.

- At any one given time, we all have cancer cells in our bodies and we rely on a healthy immune system to eliminate those cells.

Here's what we don't know:

- If a high sugar diet is maintained, and that leads to an immune system that doesn't function quite as well acutely, does that mean it doesn't function quite as well overall?
- If a high sugar diet is maintained over a long period of time, can we permanently change the efficiency of our immune system?
- Can cancer cells survive for the simple reason of there being too much sugar in the body? In other words, if cells that are supposed to be eliminated by a healthy immune system are introduced to an environment in which they can thrive in a host whose immune system isn't quite top notch, can they do so?

These are questions that many women have asked. This is a subject of hot debate amongst medical professionals, as well, for which no answers have been provided because the research is simply lacking. That simple fact alone is enough for most people to reduce their sugar intake because we simply don't know the extent of the damage that can happen with a high sugar diet.

Spicy Foods
The suggestion to cut spicy food out of your diet is purely a practical one. The findings that have been collected on spicy

food and its effect on perimenopausal and menopausal women show a close correlation with amount consumed and the incidence of hot flashes. This means that the more spicy food is eaten, the more frequent the occurrence of hot flashes becomes. Anecdotally, my own clients report this is quite true.

There are no long-term concerns about spicy food, to date, that have been presented in the research, other than possibly heartburn, but the data on that appears inconsistent. Gastric problems with spicy foods also seem to be isolated to Western populations and not a worldwide problem, which some say points to the quality of our food compared with other countries around the world. Whether that is the case or not, it seems that making spicy food a rare indulgence would be a sensible idea, perhaps especially if you reside in a Western nation.

Alcohol
Most women report that, while changing their diet may be challenging, eliminating alcohol from their diet is not and is one of the easiest steps for them to take in order to relieve their menopause symptoms.

There is ample research on alcohol and its negative effect on the liver, but how does this directly affect the menopausal woman? Well, the research shows that a liver overburdened by the consistent use of alcohol, cannot efficiently break down the hormone estrogen. Most healthcare professionals agree that two drinks a day is enough to effect the liver.[3] This can have a

---

[3] http://www.mayoclinic.com/health/alcohol/SC00024

significant effect on the menopausal woman and can aggravate or cause symptoms that may already exist.

Many women experiencing menopause report their hot flashes are aggravated by alcoholic beverages. In fact, as little as one alcoholic beverage a week has been shown to increase the occurrence of hot flashes. Many of my own clients have put this together on their own and come to me already having taken this step. Most report a reduction in their hot flashes.

Mental/emotional imbalances are also likely to worsen with the inclusion of alcohol in the diet. This can be for a few reasons. One reason would be that alcohol is a straight sugar. It's not only derived from it, it is broken back down into it once it is in the body. This can lead, as we have already discussed, to the blood sugar imbalances that can negatively effect hormone balance, causing irritability, depression, and low moods. Another reason alcohol could worsen concerns such as those aforementioned, which many menopausal women report they already struggle with, is because of its depressant nature. In some individuals, it promotes irritability and occurrences of anger as a natural side effect. This highlights the common sense conclusion that a menopausal woman already struggling with mental/emotional symptoms would do well to avoid alcohol, as to avoid a possible exacerbation of her symptoms.

Women with menopause frequently report vaginal dryness, infections, irritation, and pain during sexual activity. Any effort to keep your tissues healthy and well hydrated is not a wasted one and is very important to many women who experience

15

these symptoms during menopause. Alcohol is a very drying substance and will alter the moisture content of all the tissues in your body. Avoiding alcohol is a step in the right direction toward doing what you can to minimize this concern from happening or, if it already exists, from making it worse.

Insomnia and other sleep difficulties, commonly reported by menopausal women, are also aggravated by alcohol. Many people mistakenly associate having a glass of wine before bed with relaxation or a better sleep. Sounds nonsensical when you consider that having alcohol as little as two hours before bed can not only impact the quality of your sleep, preventing you from ever entering the precious stage of sleep called "deep sleep" we all need, but can significantly reduce the quantity of sleep you get. Many of my own clients report that when they include alcohol in their diet, they wake more frequently than they do when alcohol is not in their diet.

Weight gain is one of the most frustrating symptoms for most menopausal women. Having alcohol as a part of your regular diet will ensure that not only will you experience the weight gain that most women dread, it will be much harder for you to lose the weight. As we already discussed, alcohol is made of sugar. And we've already discussed the benefits of a low sugar diet, so there is no need to re-hash. As a take home for you to consider, though, in all my experience with my clients, their weight gain and their dieting, I have consistently seen that, in general, there is nothing as powerful as alcohol at making you gain weight. Some of my clients report that if they could repeat that night out to dinner, they would have rather had an entire second helping of their dinner rather than have that alcoholic drink because they would have had more food without as much weight to work off. These observations come with experience at watching your diet and how it affects you and your symptoms. If this isn't already natural to you, it will come to you over time as you practice doing and watching.

Future Concerns of Alcohol Consumption

Contrary to what most people may think, you don't have to be an alcoholic, recovered or otherwise, to have long standing effects on your health from alcohol.

Health experts agree that having just two drinks a day (there's that number again) is enough to increase your risk of developing high blood pressure. Of course, the more you drink, the better your odds are of developing high blood pressure, but it is clear from the research that even moderate quantities of alcohol can have a negative effect on your health over time. That isn't even where alcohol's negative potential ends. Not only do you increase your chances of having a stroke, but many other cardiovascular events, as well, even if you don't have a family history of them. This is important to menopausal women, especially. Estrogen protects women from developing heart disease by lowering your bad and total cholesterol and raising your good cholesterol. As you go through menopause, your estrogen levels decline, effectively allowing the potential reversal of this favorable cholesterol balance since you have less hormone to keep it in check. This increases a woman's cardiovascular disease risk as she goes through menopause and beyond. Doing what you can to keep the balance in your favor might just save your life, and avoiding alcohol on a regular basis, is a good first step.

Alcohol's impact still doesn't end there. The research shows that if alcohol is consumed in excess, it can lead to osteoporosis. This, of course, increases your likelihood of hip fractures, as well as other bone related problems, in the future. Not only that, since alcohol is very efficient at depleting your vitamin and mineral levels, it can contribute to a general nutritional deficiency that can lead to numerous avoidable health concerns. This is similar to what we discussed with caffeine, only much more likely, since alcohol is much more powerful than caffeine and requires more from the body in order to be used as fuel.

Refined/Processed Foods

The effect of refined and processed food on the body is profound and very similar to what we discussed with sugar. Because it is so similar, there really is no need to repeat all of the specifics of what could happen. A simple re-cap is more appropriate. If you consume refined/processed foods often, you can look forward to problems:

- Maintaining normal blood sugar levels: contributes to irritability and mood swings
- Maintaining a healthy weight: makes you more at risk for obesity, heart attacks, strokes, high blood, pressure, etc.

Perhaps the biggest question I get from my menopausal clients, and that women ask in general, is, "How often is too often?"

And the answer is that it completely depends. It depends on your body type, your metabolism, the amount you eat per indulgence, if you exercise, how often you exercise, and what exactly you are eating. Not a fair answer is it? Most people expect a cookie cutter answer such as "once a week", and are often disappointed when they adhere to the suggestion and meet failure. They fail because a suggestion like that is ludicrous when applied to the masses. Everyone is different. We all look different on the outside, so there is no reason to believe that we all operate the same way on the inside.

Your "how often" will be something you'll have to experiment with in order to come to an appropriate frequency. Once a week for most people, in my experience, is too often. And I'll tell you why ..... because on that special "cheat day", most people will lose complete control. They'll supersize everything, they'll have third helpings, they'll add a second dinner, etc. This can have an effect on everything from weight to other unpleasant symptoms of menopause like aching joints, moodiness, and low libido. If your portions were small and occurred perhaps at one meal, instead of all three, then maybe once a week might work. Some might do this and discover it is still too often. Obviously, they will get to indulge less. The more you experiment and pay attention, the more success you'll meet with. The main take away is: you don't want to do anything that's going to aggravate your symptoms and make you feel worse. So, doing what you can to keep your symptoms at bay is a good practice.

Not sure how to tell if what you're eating is refined or processed? A general rule of thumb, not a complete fail-safe mind you, is that if it comes in a box or a bag and has more than three ingredients or so, it is processed. We can go on all day about possible exceptions to this rule, like beans, raisins, or frozen veggies, but the general idea should be clear. If you need more clarification, think about the shelf life of the food. If you can put it on a shelf (refrigerated or not) and it can stay good for more than a week, it is likely processed.

Saturated Fats
Foods high in saturated fats such as bacon, sausage, processed meats, ham, butter, breaded (fried) items, baked goods, cheese, and red meat for example, will not only make a menopausal woman's battle with weight gain harder, it will increase her cardiovascular risk. This will make you more at risk for a negative cardiovascular event already discussed like strokes or high blood pressure. The research behind this is substantial and very clear. Furthermore, saturated fat has an obvious ability to cause not only negative long-term, but short-term effects.

A good example of a short-term effect is musculoskeletal concerns. I have had many a client report that when they eat more foods that are high in saturated fats (especially from meat), they notice a difference in their joints. They feel more stiff when they wake in the morning, more pain than usual, or a general sore feeling. There is some research to support the relationship between fats (especially from meat) and possible effects on the joints but the jury is still out on whether that relationship is causal or not, meaning we don't know if it actually causes negative effects on the joints. Suffice it to say though, that when people cut these saturated fats out of their diet, or reduce them greatly, many notice a tremendous positive difference in their existing musculoskeletal concerns.

Animal Protein and Animal Related Products

This last section I am going to address is a very important area of nutrition to be aware of because of the substantial and very clear benefits of omitting it, or drastically reducing it, from your regular diet.

An abundance of scientific literature has consistently demonstrated the relationship between animal protein and animal related products and disease. In the studies, it reveals how it is not enough to decrease saturated fats from the diet to see a significant difference in heart disease, other cardiovascular concerns, or even cancer. It seems that the amount of animal protein consumed shows a very strong correlation with these things, more than saturated fats do. In other words, the more animal protein is consumed, the more likely it is these diseases will develop. Here is small summary of what we know is true about the excessive intake of animal protein:

- It encourages bone loss
- It increases cholesterol
- It promotes cancer

This is particularly important and relevant to a woman going through menopause for many reasons:

- Menopause is a time during which there are many hormonal changes. These changes create significant symptoms that can be alleviated if hormonal levels are adequately controlled. Animal related products have been shown to cause hormonal abnormalities from early reproductive age and on. The fact that many animal foods are raised and manufactured with additional hormones has made this problem worse.

- Menopausal women, as already discussed, lose some natural protection against heart disease due to declining hormonal levels, putting them more at risk. A diet high in animal protein and animal related products has a direct correlation with the increased incidence of heart disease.

- As discussed above, a diet high in animal products will raise cholesterol levels making a menopausal woman's job of keeping these in check even harder.

- Since animal products are particularly rich in fats and calories, they make the job of weight loss very difficult. Weight loss is something that women going through menopause frequently struggle with.

- Menopausal women are particularly concerned with the integrity of their bones since estrogen had the job of protecting them before it started declining. Studies indicate an increased excretion of calcium from the body directly corresponds with an elevated animal protein intake. Furthermore, animal foods promote an acidic environment in the body which the body tries to offset by releasing calcium from the bones.

- Menopausal women fall in the age range where they usually start becoming more aware of their health and what they can do to optimize it. Unfortunately, that age range is also when we start seeing cancer occur more. A diet rich in animal protein does just the opposite of optimizing health by encouraging the growth of cancer. Multiple studies have shown this including the very famous The China Study, by T. Colin Campbell, Ph.D., which is the most comprehensive study ever done on the relationship between diet and disease. In it, he is able to demonstrate across multiple populations with various dietary habits the effects animal protein has on the body and how disease starts to occur more frequently in populations that have a high intake of animal foods.

Clearly, the most significant effects that animal protein and animal related products seem to have on the health of a menopausal woman are those dealing with the long term. Many of my own clients report, though, that once they omit or drastically reduce animal foods from their diet they see a positive difference in their musculoskeletal concerns, bloating, weight loss, and even low libido.

It is, of course, not required to stop eating animal protein or animal related products in order to experience a marked relief or change in your menopausal symptoms. However, according to the years of research by clinical and nutritional experts and reports from many of my own clients, the benefits are obvious and cannot be ignored. Therefore, I strongly encourage you to consider completely omitting animal protein and animal related products from your regular diet or at the very least reducing them dramatically. Not only may you see a difference in the menopausal symptoms you may be experiencing, you will lower your chronic disease and cancer risk dramatically.

Does this mean you can never have any meat or cheese? Absolutely not! Holidays would probably not be complete for most without the indulgence in the family fondeaux, meatloaf, stuffed turkey, etc. And if you really were serious about cutting out all animal protein and animal related products from your regular diet and resolved to only indulge on holidays or other such occasions, that would be ideal and you would probably not see a big flare in your symptoms (depending on how much you indulge). However, if you feel that you must have more than the occasional indulgence, having animal products once a week is the upper limit for most. After that, not only do rates for cancer and chronic disease go up, symptoms start to return.

Snapshot of What You Just Learned and Some Examples

Avoid:
- Caffeine
- Sugar: candy, ice cream, baked goods, sodas, cereals
- Spicy Foods
- Alcohol
- Refined/Processed foods: chips, frozen ready to eat meals, ready to eat meals that come in a box, fast food, breads, cookies, packaged snacks, anything with refined flour in it
- Saturated Fats: red meats, butter, full fat cheese, fried foods
- Animal Protein and Animal Related Products: red meat, chicken, cheese, eggs, milk

Client Case Study: Danielle

"I was a skeptic when it came to natural medicine. I had never really had any experience with it and didn't know anyone who did. When I started going through menopause, I did what everyone does. I read some stuff online and tried it. When that didn't work, I went to see my OBGYN. He gave me a few recommendations but nothing really seemed to change. That's when the insomnia and the night sweats started happening. Before, I was just having some minor hot flashes and fatigue that I thought would go away after a year or so. But it seemed like my body was just revving up for the main show.

For the next 6 months, every night I would go to sleep and just lie there sleepless for what seemed like hours. And when I would manage to fall asleep, I would wake up sometimes 5 times a night dripping in sweat and then lie there sleepless again once the heat would dissipate. After 3 months of this, I was starting to get extreme irritability. To add insult to injury, the hot flashes that had been minor were now graduating to major and were consuming me. Add on 3 more months of not sleeping, being hot and sweaty all night and all day, and I felt like I was going positively insane. That's when I turned to natural medicine.

After a rather long appointment, my natural health practitioner outlined a diet she wanted me to try for a few weeks. I told her I wanted to do something a little less involved and so she told me to at least stop drinking coffee and anything else that had caffeine in it. She also told me to stay away from sugar. Then, after 6 weeks, we would come back and see if I was ready for more. You may as well have chopped my arms off. I lived off of coffee and drank 6 cups of it a day. And as a journalist, you don't get very regular hours, and so sugary snacks would sometimes make my meals. But I was desperate and willing to try anything.

I started following all her instructions and after 2 weeks, I noticed my hot flashes were 30% less! I got very excited about that and continued to follow her plan. After 3 and a half weeks, my night sweats were only happening once a night now and I was able to sleep a good 5 hours straight, whereas before I was only getting 3 hours of sleep. Moreover, my hot flashes were steadily continuing to decrease. I was becoming a happy camper. 5 weeks into her plan, my night sweats had disappeared and although I was still not falling asleep right away I would only lie there for 45 minutes until I would finally drift off and stay asleep for a solid 7 hours.

6 weeks after I started my journey, it was time for my follow up. Night sweats? Gone. Insomina? 90% better. Hot flashes? 75% better. When my natural health practitioner asked me if I was ready to try more, I told her I was pretty much going to do whatever she told me to. I hadn't felt this good in a long time. It was hard for me to believe that just staying away from those two things could help me feel this good. Can you imagine if I did more? I am completely won over by my natural medicine practitioner and what natural medicine is capable of. Do

yourself a favor and try this route first. I wish that I hadn't wasted so much time with all the other stuff."

-Danielle*, 56 years old
Austin, Texas

Step 2: Foods To Eat More Of

Identify Foods That Can Pave The Way To Helping You Feel Better

With the bad news out of the way, we can now focus on all the food you do get to eat. This step is a lot more fun, and way more inclusive. The foods we'll discuss are all parts of a symbiotic whole. They will work together to:

- Lower your cardiovascular risk of negative events
- Keep your blood sugar and blood pressure low
- Create a nutrient rich environment that will preserve your bones: protect you from osteoporosis and fractures
- Enhance your immunity by boosting your vitamin and mineral status
- Keep your moods even
- Prevent weight gain
- Enhance your brain health: boosting memory and focus

In general, here is what you should focus most of your dietary attention on:

29

- Vegetables
- Fruits
- Beans and Legumes
- Nuts and Seeds
- Whole Grains (optional)
- Cold-Water Fish (optional)
- Oils (optional)

And you should focus on them more or less in that order. You're going to want to know why this is, of course. Let's dive into it going into each bullet point briefly to give you a small summary of the benefits they will provide to you.

Vegetables

These can be eaten raw or cooked and I encourage you to eat *__as much as you want__* of both! (Isn't it nice that you can have an unlimited quantity of something?) Here's why:

- You just can't overdo it when you eat these because they have too much fiber in them to allow you to go beyond what your stomach can hold.
- They don't stay in your gut very long, which promotes weight loss.
- They have a very low impact on your blood glucose level, which promotes steady blood glucose levels. This will help you to avoid mood swings, irritability, and other mental/emotional symptoms that may accompany menopause.

- They have a high amount of anti-oxidant potential and vitamin/mineral content in them that can help strengthen your immune system both short and long term.
- Their high vitamin/mineral content can also have a tremendous positive impact on your memory and cognitive function.
- If your diet is founded in vegetables and other plant based proteins, it is unlikely you will have to deal with cardiovascular disease and blood pressure problems.
- They have a high mineral content that can reinforce the integrity and strength of your bones, helping you to avoid fractures and breaks in the future.

There are some vegetables that you'll want to stay away from for the most part if you already have blood sugar problems or struggle with weight gain. These would include the high starch vegetables such as: potatoes (sweet and white), yams, pumpkin, squashes (winter, butternut and acorn), parsnips, corn (considered a grain by most now), and both regular and water chestnuts. If you neither have blood sugar problems nor struggle with weight gain, you can include the aforementioned in your diet if you wish. But really try and stick to greener veggies and veggies with more color since they provide a much higher nutritional value to your diet and your life.

It is also wise to stay away from canned veggies, as their salt content tends to be high and their nutritional value very low. Frozen veggies, however, are just fine and the person who invented that idea should be celebrated often! They make a nice and easy addition to your diet because you can store what you don't need and save it for later, instead of eating it all right away. You can see a list of recommended veggies in the snapshot section at the end of this step.

Fruits

Fruit has gotten a bad reputation lately. Perhaps it is because of their naturally high sugar content, or fad diets touting that they are the enemy in the battle against weight loss (not necessarily true by the way). Whatever the case may be, fruit should not be ignored and is an important part of a nutrient rich diet that has the potential to offer you beneficial relief from menopausal symptoms. I recommend that you eat up to 3-4 servings of fresh or frozen fruits daily and here is why:

- Fresh or frozen, many fruits are packed with antioxidants and phytonutrients that can enhance your short and long term immunity. This can protect you and make you less likely to get common colds, viruses, even cancer.
- Berries, in particular, have been shown to be beneficial in preventing cardiovascular disease and any related events. This is important for women in their menopausal years.
- Many fruits have been shown to contain antioxidants that have a positive impact on the areas of the brain responsible for memory and learning.
- They make an easy and wholesome breakfast that can take less than 5 minutes to prepare, taking the thought out of "cooking".
- A diet rich in veggies and fruits and low in saturated fats, grains, and processed foods can be the key to alleviating

symptoms of not just menopause, but chronic diseases for which we have no cure.

Canned fruit is not as nutritious as fresh or frozen and often has added sweeteners. Therefore, I recommend you stay away from it. A popular trend recently is to juice fruits and add them to veggies in a breakfast smoothie. While this is better than a stack of pancakes, it can be very easy to lose track of how much fruit you put in your smoothie, making it easy to eat too many. Plus, you lose out on the fiber that is in the fresh or frozen fruit making the nutrient value of your smoothie lower than if you were just to eat the whole fruit. This means less benefit for you. I recommend you stick to eating the fruit in its fresh or frozen form to get the most benefit from your food. The last thing you'll want to stay away from is dried fruit for two reasons: it is very high in sugar and easy to get carried away with eating too much of it since it is usually small in size. You can see a list of recommended fruits in the snapshot section at the end of this step.

Beans and Legumes

This is perhaps my favorite food to recommend. They are easy to find, easy to prepare, and even easier to eat. I recommend you eat a lot of these and quite often. Most people can't eat very many in one sitting because they are particularly filling, but if you need a serving size limit for weight loss purposes, try not to eat more than a cup and a half cooked or so throughout the whole day. If weight is not an issue, then feel free to have more. Most people recommend much less than that because they are concerned about the calories they contain. I think that if your diet is rich in beans and legumes (plant proteins) and not in animal protein and animal related products, then you can have much more of them. Here is why beans and legumes are awesome additions to your diet:

- They can be extremely versatile: hot, cold, seasoned, unseasoned, sprouted, or cooked.
- It doesn't take very much to fill you and you stay full longer: supports weight loss efforts if that is something you are struggling with during menopause.
- Studies done on them indicate they lower cholesterol and triglycerides, which can protect you from cardiovascular related events like strokes and heart attacks.
- They protect your brain and its function because they are high in B vitamins, which are necessary for proper brain health. This will protect you from age related memory concerns, dementia, and other cognitive decline issues.
- They are packed with calcium and magnesium, which can enhance the integrity of your bones, protecting you from osteoporosis in the future. If you are worried about phytate levels in your beans (substances which can interfere with calcium absorption), just soak your beans for a few hours and then cook them in fresh water. This should reduce phytate levels nicely.
- They help maintain steady blood sugar levels. This supports your mental/emotional well being, making mood swings and irritability related to menopause less likely. An added benefit to steady blood sugar levels is that you're less likely to have cravings for sweets and salty snacks.

- Soy has been demonstrated in the research to significantly reduce the occurrence and severity of hot flashes, as well as night sweats and vaginal dryness.

You can see a list of recommended beans and legumes in the snapshot section at the end of this step.

Nuts and Seeds
Nuts and seeds are a great addition to any diet, but are particularly beneficial for women going through menopause. A woman's cardiovascular disease or negative event (like a heart attack or stroke) risk goes up after we go through menopause, as we've already discussed. Therefore, anything we can do to reverse that risk would behoove us. Nuts and seeds are important to eat because:

- They have a tremendous amount of fat, but studies have shown that those fats are the healthy kind, such as omega-3, and have significant benefits to your cardiovascular health by helping lower cholesterol and decreasing your risk for a heart attack.
- They can fortify your long-term immunity and studies show that they are helpful in protecting you against cancer.
- Even a small amount will fill you and you'll stay full longer: supports weight loss efforts if this is something you struggle with during your menopause, as already discussed.

Nuts and seeds may be high in healthy fats, but they are also high in calories. If weight gain is something you are struggling with during your menopause, you should really only eat about ¼ cup per day. If weight is not an issue for you, feel free to ignore this limit. A note on flaxseeds: they should be ground if you are to derive any benefit from them, otherwise, they will just be passed. They should also be refrigerated so the natural oils in them will be preserved.

One last note on nuts and seeds: they should be eaten raw. Most grocery stores offer nuts and seeds pre-packaged, which is a problem because they are usually cooked, roasted, or baked in some kind of fatty oil or worse, salt and sugar are added to them. It is right there in the ingredient label, if you doubt this. Make sure what you are getting is only the raw nut or seed. You can see a list of recommended nuts and seeds in the snapshot section at the end of this step.

<u>Whole Grains (Optional)</u>
It has been my experience that this group of food is often very misunderstood. There has been lots of media lately about how whole grain bread is a better choice for you than your common white bread. There are hundreds of variations on this from whole grain tortillas, whole grain cereals, whole grain bagels, even whole grain pancakes. And while the whole grain version of anything might have a slightly higher nutritional profile than the non-whole grain version, no one has paused to mention the obvious: that even if you are consuming a whole grain version of something, you are still eating a refined and processed food. This can lead, as we've already discussed, to unstable blood

sugar levels, irritability, depression, osteoporosis, insomnia, cardiovascular problems, etc. This is not a good consequence for a woman going through menopause.

What should be focused on is the consumption of **_only_** whole grains, not processed foods with whole grains in them. You can see a list of recommended whole grains in the snapshot section at the end of this step.

You'll notice there isn't a list of benefits for this option. That's because there really aren't any significant benefits of this group of food to menopausal women and their symptoms. And if you really want to know the truth, any grain-based diet, even a whole grain one, will not provide you with the nutritional bedrock you need in order to decrease any menopausal symptoms you may be experiencing, nor will it help you to avoid the common health problems many menopausal women face in the future. Seeing as grains play a large part in the diet of many, though, it is important to address the whole grain issue so we can separate fact from fiction.

I recommend you stay away from grains entirely if you struggle with weight loss or blood sugar issues. Eating grains will not help you to win either battle in any way, shape, or form. If you do not struggle with either one of these problems, then feel free to make this option as frequent as you choose.

Cold-Water Fish (Optional)
We've already discussed the potential risk that animal protein can pose to a menopausal woman. However, if you are going

to choose to include some animal protein in your diet, reach for cold-water fish instead. These are going to provide you with some beneficial fats that may promote your cardiovascular health.

It is important to be aware of where your fish comes from and to stay away from fish that has a high mercury content, as mercury is extremely toxic to the body and causes a whole host of problems that are not the subject of this book. It is also important to be aware of the fact that studies do not indicate any increased cardiovascular or other health benefit to including fish more than once or twice a week in your diet.[4]

Stay away from farm raised fish or fish that doesn't specify where it was caught. You are going to want to concentrate on wild caught fish since those fish are usually from oceans that don't have high concentrations of dangerous toxins, aren't overharvested, and have higher levels of beneficial fats in them.

You will notice, once again, the absence of a list of benefits. That is because, while cold-water fish can provide some benefit, they aren't very significant to the menopausal woman. This food should be treated like the whole grains section above it: have it if you wish but be aware that it offers little actual benefit to the menopause symptoms you may be experiencing. Therefore, it is optional. You can see a list of recommended cold-water fish in the snapshot section at the end of this step.

---

[4] http://www.hsph.harvard.edu/nutritionsource/fish/

Oils (Optional)

This last section is important for you to know about rather than it is about me recommending you include it in your diet. Cooking oils are often used in cooking, baking, and for creating dressings and sauces. It is important to be aware that most cooking oils commonly used can pose a risk to your cardiovascular health as well as increase the amount of calories you consume. We've already discussed the cardiovascular health issue for menopausal women, so there is no need to re-hash.

Healthier oil choices like coconut and olive oil are much better substitutes for your typical canola, sunflower, corn, palm, or sesame oil, not to mention butter, margarine, or worse, shortening. Coconut and olive oil are better choices because they are among the few that possess significant benefits. Sure, there are others like hemp, flax, pumpkin seed, almond, pecan, and even macadamia. However, most traditional stores won't carry these at all or will have a limited supply of those just mentioned and they tend to be very expensive. This guide is about giving you options you can find anywhere even if you don't have access to a super exclusive "health food" store. I don't want to blow your mind with what you could include that may work, but rather introduce you to what you should include that will likely benefit you. You can achieve more benefit for less dollar with coconut and olive oil.

Coconut oil is high in good saturated fats that have proven to be beneficial, as well as in anti-viral properties that have the potential to enhance your immune system. It should be purchased unrefined and in virgin form. Olive oil is high in flavonoids and monosaturated fats, which are the good kind of fat. It should also be in unrefined and virgin or extra virgin form.

Olive oil will the best oil choice if you are looking to lower your cholesterol levels, lose weight, and even just enhance the flavor of your food. Take note that it is pretty high in calories, though. So, don't drizzle it generously as it will add up over time. Rather, use it sparingly. A couple of tablespoons a day or less is a good limit if you struggle with weight gain. If not, you can have more.

I hesitate to recommend coconut oil for the simple reason that it is high in saturated fat. (It is also quite high in calories, but that is not necessarily what concerns me.) Even if those fats are beneficial, this will not be a good choice for those who need to lose weight, get blood sugar problems under control, lower cholesterol levels, or minimize their risk for heart disease. It makes no sense to pile fat on any of the aforementioned conditions. Therefore, if you have one of them and still want to use cooking oil, olive oil will be your best bet.

Once again, you will notice no list of benefits for this section! There really aren't any that are significant to the health of a menopausal woman and that is what makes this section optional. Remember that oils, even the ones I have just offered as recommendations, are not "health foods" and won't build the good foundation necessary for a strong immune system, increased quality of life, or to conquer menopausal symptoms.

If you are going to include oils in your diet, though, make it one of the recommended ones we have discussed above.

Snapshot of What You Just Learned and Some Examples

Eat More:

- Vegetables: fresh or frozen, as well as cooked. Feel free to have as many as you like. Eat **lots of** romaine lettuce, carrots, snow peas, cucumbers, tomatoes, kale, collard greens, broccoli, string beans, peas, cauliflower, asparagus, zucchini, radishes, artichokes, Brussels sprouts, bok choy, dandelion greens, spinach, bell peppers, mushrooms, onions, celery, eggplant, and any other greens. If you struggle with blood sugar problems or weight loss, **avoid**: potatoes (sweet and white), yams, pumpkin, squashes (winter, butternut and acorn), parsnips, corn, and both regular and water chestnuts. Avoid canned veggies.

- Fruits: fresh or frozen. Enjoy up to 3-4 servings of fruit: blueberries, blackberries, raspberries, strawberries, (any berry!), oranges, apples, pears, grapes, lemons, limes, plums, peaches, kiwi, cherries, mangoes, papaya, kumquats, pomegranates, apricots, avocadoes, dragon fruit, melons, watermelon, and pineapples. A serving would be one cup. Avoid canned and dried fruit.

- Beans and Legumes: pinto beans, black beans, red beans, lentils, split peas, soybeans, garbanzo beans, edamame, black-eyed peas, and white beans. Tofu would go here, as well. Enjoy up to one cup and a half cups of cooked beans or legumes if you need to lose weight. If not, enjoy more.

- <u>Nuts and Seeds</u>: walnuts, almonds, cashews, pecans, macadamias, pistachios, sesame seeds, sunflower seeds, hemp seeds, flaxseeds, chia seeds, and pumpkin seeds. If you struggle with weight loss, eat only ¼ cup. Otherwise, enjoy more. Remember to focus on finding them raw.
- <u>Whole Grains (optional)</u>: brown rice, quinoa, and steel cut oats.
- <u>Cold-Water Fish (optional)</u>: salmon, herring, halibut, and sardines. Yes, tuna and mackerel are cold-water fish but these are rather high in mercury, which is toxic as already discussed. Therefore, avoid these.
- <u>Oils (optional)</u>: Olive oil and coconut oil. Up to two tablespoons per day if you need to lose weight.

Client Case Study: Olivia

"I had been going to my GP for 2 years for really bad mood swings and depression that started when I turned 50. He told me it was menopause and wrote a never-ending stream of prescriptions for adrenal this or thyroid that. Nothing seemed to help much and I noticed that after a year, I started to gain weight but I hadn't changed anything about my diet. Still, I stuck with the meds in the hope that they would just kick in one day. 40 pounds later and still feeling blue, I decided to give alternative medicine a try.

When I went, I wasn't really expecting to hear that my diet needed to change and was probably responsible for a lot of my symptoms. No one had ever asked me about anything related to my diet so I had no clue that it could be making me feel worse. I was given very detailed instructions about a new way of eating and told to come back in 7 weeks. I hated diets and thought this was going to be an epic failure. And honestly, didn't see the relationship to my symptoms. But I liked that I could eat real food and didn't have to do anything weird with meal replacement shakes or supplements that tasted nasty. Besides, I figured that I had nothing to lose.

After 2 weeks, I had lost 12 pounds. I also noticed that my mood swings, although they were still happening, were not happening as often and were not as severe. I was elated! It was nice to lose weight, but honestly I was more excited about my mood swings because I hadn't seen any change in them in the last couple of years. And so, I kept at it. After 4 weeks, I had lost 19 pounds, but that wasn't the really good part. My depression was starting to lift. I would have whole days where it didn't happen at all. And my mood swings would only happen once a week now. After 6 weeks, I had lost 25 pounds and was feeling like a whole new person. No moods swings at all were happening now and what I was calling 'depression' had been gone for a whole week. At my follow up visit at 7 weeks, I was nothing short of giddy. My natural health practitioner was almost startled at my transformation and encouraged me to continue doing what I was doing.

Now 7 months later, I feel like I have a new lease on life. The 'depression' is still gone, the mood swings don't happen anymore (unless I misbehave and eat something I'm not supposed to). I am also now 55 pounds lighter than I was when I first started alternative medicine, and am actually at a normal weight for my height. That hasn't happened since I was 27 years old!

If anyone is going through a menopause like the one I was going through, I encourage them to try alternative medicine sooner rather than later. I couldn't believe the difference it made in my life. My only regret is that I didn't start it sooner."

-Olivia*, 53 years old
San Antonio, Texas

Step 3: Exercise

See How Half An Hour Can Change Your Life

This step will be short and sweet because of its straightforward nature. Step 3 is devoted to exercise. After reading this step you will know:

- How exercise can benefit a woman going through menopause
- How often you need to do it in order to benefit
- The exercise that is the most important (and probably the one you're not doing!)

Before you scoff, roll your eyes, and skip this step entirely, consider this: women who exercise regularly experience 65% less hot flashes than women who don't exercise regularly.[5] And their hot flashes don't last as long when they do get them and they're not as intense! This is enough to get even the most stubborn of my clients to at least take the scenic route to their mailbox.

---

[5] http://www.fhcrc.org/content/dam/public/Treatment-Suport/survivorship/Healthy-Links/Menopausal%20Symptoms.pdf

Exercise can also benefit women going through menopause in many other ways:

- Makes weight loss easier: reducing that stubborn belly fat so many women going through menopause talk about
- Helps you fall asleep faster and stay asleep longer: reducing insomnia and night waking
- Gives you more energy that lasts throughout the day: battling that eternal fatigue women report can be the bane of their existence
- Boosts short term memory function and other cognitive abilities: women frequently report that their memory is significantly impacted upon entering menopause, leaving them confused and frightened
- Alleviates anxiety and depression symptoms: these are common concerns that often accompany, women frequently report, the beginning of menopause
- Boosts good cholesterol while reducing bad cholesterol: protecting menopausal women from heart disease, stroke, and high blood pressure.
- Is the only way to build bone: protecting women from osteoporosis

What And How Much Exercise Should You Be Doing?

Of course, the benefits don't end there, but these are the most relevant to the woman going through menopause. The next question I get is usually a practical one: "What should I do for exercise?" The answer is: Absolutely anything you want. There is not one form of exercise more superior to another and that is the absolute truth. Your body doesn't comprehend the difference between different forms of exercise, per se. All it does perceive are the benefits of increased circulation, toned body parts allowing easier and stronger movements, more oxygen being delivered to the muscles and the tissues, and increased levels of chemicals that benefit brain health.

Big tip: Make sure you choose something you actually enjoy. If you hate the elliptical or any other fitness machine, please avoid a gym and its membership. Pick something you will actually look forward to doing the next time you do it. And if you need several different forms of exercise to prevent you from getting bored, then no problem! Keep alternating them and even alternate the days you do them on to provide the maximum benefit. Any form of exercise is going to benefit you physically, but this next bit of information is extra important because it involves the brain. Whatever you do choose to do, make sure that it provides you both cardiovascular exercise and resistance training. A substantial amount of medical research points to the combination of the two being the best prevention against cognitive decline.

Any exercise is better than no exercise at all, and everyone has different needs so the frequency of exercise recommended will differ for everyone. In general, though, 30-45 minutes 3-4 times a week is associated with the best results physically, mentally, and emotionally for most.

The Most Important Exercise You're Not Doing
If you already have a regular fitness routine, good for you! But chances are high that you are leaving the most important part of

your body out of your fitness regime: your brain. It turns out your superior thinking organ needs exercise, too. There is ample evidence supporting how important it is to engage the brain to prevent dementia, Alzheimer's disease, and other cognitive related decline. Basically the old adage, "Use it or lose it" applies here.

There are many things you can do to exercise your brain and keep it sharp. And it won't only benefit your long-term brain health, it will enhance your short-term brain health as well. In any "brain exercise" routine, the objective is do new things that engage different parts of the brain so that new connections are formed between the neurons. These new connections are important because they help you to retain information, which is the foundation of the learning process. Basically, don't stop learning. This can apply to anything and everything, which is a pretty broad recommendation. So here are some ideas that are practical and that have shown success:

- Learn a new language: American Sign Language, Spanish, Chinese
- Take up a new hobby: knitting, photography, art
- Acquire a new skill: woodworking, beekeeping, remodeling
- Read new books: in different genres than your usual ones
- Travel: to new places in particular so you can encounter the unfamiliar
- Crosswords, puzzles, games, Sudoku: Good old brain teasers. These games were once the mainstay for

people looking to keep their brains sharp. Although we're not sure if they provide as much protection from cognitive decline as we thought, they still make the brain work and keep it thinking as long as you do new games each time. And that still translates to some benefit.

- Brain training: I have listed this as an option because the online presence of the companies that offer these types of services is extremely pervasive, and they are very good at promoting their benefits. This perhaps explains their exponential growth over the past 5 years or so. However, the research behind the use of these types of services for actually preventing cognitive related decline and memory loss is lacking, at best, and there needs to be much more of it to prove the worth of (and your investment into) these services. That's not to say that tools like these won't benefit you at all. However, medical experts believe they may not provide as much protection as they are portrayed to offer. Still, if this is something you are eager to try, a simple Internet search will uncover many options for you.

There really is no recommended frequency or amount of "brain exercise" because the more you do, the more benefit you will gain. The exercise does need to be consistent, though, in order for the brain to experience the most benefit.

Client Case Study: Gertrude

"I am an amateur natural medicine enthusiast and I maintain a pretty healthy diet. So when I started getting hot flashes, I naturally turned to alternative medicine to help me. My hot flashes were only happening about 5 or 6 times a day, but I didn't want them to get overwhelming like I had read they could get. So, I took everything that I read about to help me feel better. Vitamins, herbs, even exotic natural remedies. You name it, I took it. And I really thought that with a little bit of luck, I might come across at least one thing that would make a dent in my hot flashes. But absolutely nothing worked. And to make matters worse, my hot flashes were starting to increase to about 10 times a day. This went on for a year before I went to go see Cristina.

By that time, I was fed up with natural medicine and was actually considering some sort of hormonal therapy. Because I was in such a sensitive space, Cristina recommended something much more fundamental than her usual. She told me I needed to start exercising. I cringed. I loved natural medicine and had been using it for years, but I hated to exercise. I also couldn't believe that something that simple could unlock any kind of relief for me. I was desperate though, and so I decided that I would head down to a nearby community pool to see what would happen.

I started doing laps for 30 minutes every day and after 2 weeks, started noticing a difference in my symptoms. I noticed that my

51

hot flashes were actually starting to lessen in the afternoons! I couldn't believe that it was the exercise, but it was the only thing I had changed and so I stopped doing it to see what would happen. That was a very bad decision. Not only did my hot flashes start to escalate after 5 days, but it seemed like they had gotten hotter! I threw myself in the pool after that, and thankfully they decreased by about 50%.

As I started my follow up visits, Cristina pointed out the holes in my diet that I needed to clean up and started homeopathic medicine with me as well. Slowly but surely, after about 12 weeks, my hot flashes went away. It's been a year and a half now, and I feel better than ever. I am hot flash free except when I spend long periods of time, like holidays, away from the pool. But thankfully, I know how to fix that now."

-Gertrude*, 56 years old
Austin, Texas

Step 4: Common Homeopathic Remedies

Uncover Natural Medicine's Best Kept Secret For Symptom Relief

The last step is the one that most menopausal women seem to have no compliance issue with. Even though it is the last step in this short guide, it is a very powerful one. And one that can work what some of my own clients call "miracles" **without** ever having to do any of the other steps. Be that as it may, I invite you to experience and appreciate the benefits which can come from leading a healthy lifestyle. That *starts* with steps 1-3, and *may include* step 4.

If you feel you need to ease into these steps or just want to take it one step at a time, then this is probably the step you will want to start with. Natural medicine can encompass many therapies such as traditional Chinese medicine, acupuncture, herbal medicine, supplements, homeopathic medicine, and hydrotherapy among others. I am going to focus on the therapy that I have seen work the most consistently: homeopathic medicine.

At the end of this step you will know:

- What homeopathic medicine is and why it is so effective
- Which homeopathic remedies are the most successful for symptoms of menopause
- How to pick a homeopathic remedy correctly

What Is Homeopathic Medicine?

Homeopathic medicine is a system that uses very small doses of remedies. These remedies are prepared from various plants, minerals, and animal substances found in nature. This is the part that becomes counterintuitive. A homeopathic practitioner will select a remedy that causes the symptoms you are experiencing in a healthy individual, adhering to the core principle of the system, "like cures like". The idea is that if it can cause these symptoms in a healthy individual, it can eliminate them in a sick individual. For instance, if one drinks coffee they may feel fidgety, anxious, have racing thoughts, have an increased heart rate, and trouble sleeping. If you happened to have these symptoms at night because you suffered from insomnia with anxiety, a homeopathic dose of the remedy *Coffea crudum* (coffee) might help reduce and/or eliminate your symptoms.

It is these small doses, or micro-doses, of remedies that stimulate your system to heal from within, potentially alleviating symptoms you may be experiencing. Because they are administered in such small doses, they are considered extremely safe to use with everyone, including infants and pregnant women. Even though homeopathic medicine has been in use since the early 1800's with thousands of successful cases documented, there continues to be consistent research today supporting nearly two centuries of homeopathic practice with hundreds of clinical studies published in modern and respected medical journals that are too numerous to list here. I will instead point you to a resource, if the research is something that you are particularly interested in reading: http://nationalcenterforhomeopathy.org.

How This Guide Should Be Used

I've created this guide, particularly this section, to help you manage the discomforts of a normal menopause. While that will vary from woman to woman, if your symptoms are severe or ongoing, you should consult your health care professional immediately. With some exceptions, (such as but not limited to severe menstrual bleeding, blinding headaches, uncontrollable anxiety, and suicidal depression) you can safely manage your symptoms yourself if they are relatively minor. For more serious or long-term problems, it is always best practice to consult a trained homeopathic practitioner and your doctor.

It would be impossible to list every possible homeopathic remedy that could help alleviate the symptoms that so often occur during menopause. I have, instead, compiled a sampling of the most common homeopathic remedies used most often for women going through menopause.

Around 89% of my clients with menopause started their homeopathic care on one of these listed remedies and 94% of them experienced significant relief from their symptoms at their first follow up appointment four weeks later. Most, if not all, of these remedies can be found at most health food stores in a 30C potency, which is what most of my clients start with.

Once you select a remedy, take two or three pellets and let them dissolve under your tongue. Now wait to see if there is any change in your symptoms. If there is improvement, this is fantastic! You do not need to take any more doses of your homeopathic remedy. If you feel better for a while but your symptoms return, then you can take another dose of your remedy. You can continue repeating dosing your remedy as needed as long as it is helping you. If there is no improvement in your symptoms, however, either initially or upon repeated dosing, do not continue taking the remedy. You can try to choose another remedy and see if this helps you. If this doesn't work, then it is time to consult a homeopathic professional.

How To Pick A Homeopathic Remedy

Allow me to orient you to the layout of the following list of remedies and how they should be selected. The name of the remedy is in bold type and is underlined. What follows after that is a brief summary of the type of symptoms someone needing that remedy would experience during menopause. Then, there is a section labeled, 'General'. This is a description of general characteristics someone may have that makes that remedy choice much more likely. An example of this would be a desire for vinegar and sweets.

Overall, if the description of symptoms and the general characteristics match what you are experiencing, then this remedy might be the correct one for you and would be a good place to start. Though it would be nice if both sections described you exactly, they often don't, and thankfully don't need to. What is most important to focus on is the nature of your symptoms. For instance, it's important if your hot flashes move upward and are mainly in your upper body and face, as opposed to whether or not you long for vinegar and sweets. Make sure your symptoms are the main focus when selecting a remedy. For best results, use only one remedy at a time, that way if you experience improvement, you know which one the correct one is.

Most Common Homeopathic Remedies For Menopause

Sepia: sudden, frequent, hot flushes at menopause preceded by weakness and anxiety, followed by perspiration and great tendency to faint; heat starts low and moves upward; poor memory; flushes of heat are mainly in the face followed by redness; dwells on past disagreeable occurrences; mentally weak, confusing words; everything is mentally demanding; yellow brownish color to skin across the nose and cheeks; constipation; urging to urinate and involuntary urination especially at night; great dryness of the vagina; wakes up with violent beating of heart; clumsy; sleeplessness at night especially after 3 AM; as if hot water was poured on her.

General: chilly; worse from cold and in afternoon; better from vigorous exercise and warmth; indifferent attitude even to loved ones; irritable and offended easily; critical and intolerant of contradiction; sensitive to music and noise; desire for vinegar and sweets.

Sulphur: feels too hot and flushes of heat move upward; very forgetful and thinking is difficult; top of head hot; lips dry, bright red, and burning; heat and burning in face with flushing; hot flushes during menopause with hot head, hands, and feet followed by great faintness in stomach; feels suffocated and wants doors and windows open at night; flushes of heat throughout chest with heaviness, followed by heat rising to head; burning in soles and hands at night; frequent waking at night with heat, anxiety, and restlessness; difficulty falling asleep with sweat and itchy skin; frequent flushes or violent boiling throughout entire body; strong smelling sweat; itching and burning skin worse from scratching and heat.

General: very hot; worse from heat, morning, and standing; better in open air and sweating; irritable and depressed; quarrelsome and impatient; critical; sensitive to odors; thirsty and dry.

Pulsatilla: feels insane during menopause; puffy face that is red with frequent flushes; as if urine were impossible to delay; involuntary urination at night; heavy blood flow during menopause; vaginal discharge and itchiness at menopause; wakes frequently; sleeplessness from an anxious sensation of heat; intolerable burning heat at night; burning hands; attacks of flushes of heat; internal heat without external heat; one sided perspiration on head and scalp.

General: worse from warmth and in evening; better in cold and open air; cries easily; contradictory; thirstless; sensitive; symptoms change constantly; better from consolation.

Phosphorus: burning sensation as if a flame seemed to be passing through her, especially at night; feeling of intense heat running up the back; great lowness of spirits; loss of memory; brain feels tired; anxious about many things especially for others; fear something will happen; flow of thoughts difficult to arrange; lacks willpower to undertake anything; heat comes from spine; experiences burning heat in face and hands, followed by redness of cheeks and anxiety; flushes from the least emotion; tension over bladder region; burning in urinary tract with frequent urging to urinate; flushes all over beginning in hands which causes frequent waking; profuse perspiration at night during sleep on head and hands that is followed by chills.

General: worse from cold and mental exertion; oversensitive to noise, light, odors; sympathetic; fears thunderstorms; thirst for very cold water; craves ice cream.

Conium: memory weak and unable to sustain any mental effort; forgetful with excessive difficulty of recollecting things especially dates; top of head unusually hot; heat of face; sore sensation in uterus region; muscular weakness especially of lower limbs; hot flushes or sweat on dropping to sleep through the whole body; great heat internally and externally with great nervousness; most profuse sweat on head and upper body.

General: aversion to people; dwells on the past; sensitive to noise.

Calcarea carbonica: sweats easily and during sleep; easy, cold perspiration about the head, hands, and feet; apprehensive; forgetful with anxiety and palpitation; misplaces words and has a tendency to express herself wrongly; despairing and hopeless of ever getting well; heavy blood flow during menopause; restless at night with a dry heat but with cold sweat on the head, neck, and chest; frequent flushes with anxious palpitation followed by chill and cold hands; frequent attacks of sudden general heat as if she had been drenched with hot water; will sweat even if its cold.

Magnesia carbonica: irritability and restlessness; burning during urination; sleeplessness from anxious uneasiness and internal heat with great dread; whole body feels tired and

60

painful; great internal heat at night with night sweats but has an aversion to uncovering; one sided heat on right side with burning and redness of head.

Lachesis: flushes of heat and rushes of blood; weakness of whole body in the morning on rising; great physical and mental weakness; during heat, must loosen clothes around the neck because there is a sensation they inhibit the circulation of blood with a feeling of suffocation; weakness of memory and makes mistakes in writing and speaking; violent burning during urination; menopausal troubles with palpitations, flushes of heat, hemorrhages, headaches at the top of the head, and fainting spells; during menopause has flashes of heat all day and cold flashes on retiring at night; prolapse of uterus during menopause; heavy bleeding and chills at night and flushes of heat by day; persistent bloated feeling during menopause; nightly burning in palms and soles; sleeplessness from anxiety and internal restlessness; hot flushes on top of head or in hands and feet at night accompanied by great headache; perspiration hot and around neck; profuse sweat that wakes her up at night.

General: worse from sleep, heat, and tight clothes; better in open air, from cold drinks, and loosening clothes; for women who have never felt well since starting menopause, even if it has been years.

Client Case Study: Belinda

"I had been suffering with extreme menopausal symptoms for 5 years before I turned to natural medicine. I had hot flashes, night sweats, anxiety, and was extremely irritable. I might have been able to manage it all if my hot flashes weren't so severe. I would basically have a hot flash every 10 minutes...... waking and sleeping. It would start from below and move up to my face. Just before it would happen, I would get this strange feeling like something really horrible was going to happen and when it was done, I was drenched in an embarrassing sweat all over my body and my face was bright red. Because it was happening so often and had been going on for so long, I was starting to feel exhausted and weak. It was starting to interfere with my career, my life, and my relationships, so I was willing to try just about anything to see if it would help me.

I can't believe I didn't turn to it sooner. Cristina spent almost 2 hours with me at my first visit, during which she asked lots of strange questions that I thought had nothing to do with my symptoms. She also encouraged me to change my diet and exercise, but I wasn't interested in doing that because I didn't want to invest a whole lot of time and energy into things that I felt might not help me. She agreed that I needed to see improvement with something else first in order to consider diet and exercise and so we started with homeopathy. She gave me a homeopathic remedy called Sepia, which I took daily for 4 weeks. At that point, I was supposed to follow up with her. But

I didn't follow up for about 3 months because my hot flashes disappeared!

There was a difference almost immediately. The first 3 days or so, my hot flashes at night stopped happening and I was actually able to sleep through the night for the first time in years. During the day, my hot flashes were still happening but they weren't as severe and my face wasn't turning red anymore. By the end of a week, the daytime flashes were reduced to about half of what they were and the night ones were still gone. By the second week, I actually had energy and was feeling alive again. The anxiety I was getting before my hot flashes was starting to go away and by the end of the second week, wasn't happening anymore. It wasn't until the end of the third week, when I was at dinner with some co-workers on a patio outside on a summer night, that I realized I hadn't had a hot flash all day. And things have stayed that way ever since.

I really didn't see the need to keep my follow up visit because I was feeling so much better, and so I cancelled it. The only reason I went back 3 months later was to get a re-fill of my beloved homeopathic remedy, Sepia. During that follow up visit, I related to Cristina that I was almost mad at myself for not trying natural medicine sooner. I could have avoided all those years of sleeplessness and suffering. I am happy as a clam now, though. And I frequently recommend homeopathy to all my friends and colleagues going through menopause since it helped me so much. I didn't even know homeopathic medicine existed before. Now, I am officially a firm believer."

-Belinda*, 52 years old
San Antonio, Texas

About The Author

Cristina Villa Cantu is an alternative medicine practitioner with a special focus in homeopathic medicine.

She received her doctorate in Naturopathic Medicine from Southwest College of Naturopathic Medicine & Health Sciences in Tempe, Arizona. Prior to naturopathic medical school, she received her Bachelor of Science in Biology, magna cum laude, from the University of the Incarnate Word in San Antonio, Texas.

She now practices in Texas with a particular focus in women's and children's health.

After seeing the positive and irrefutable impact of naturopathic medicine on clients during her naturopathic clinical training, she became an advocate of natural therapeutics that offer effective, gentle, and safe alternatives to address health concerns and promote optimal health and wellness.

For more information, visit: www.justnaturalremedies.com.

About Naturopathic Medicine

Naturopathic medicine concentrates on whole-client wellness; the medicine is tailored to the client and emphasizes prevention and self-care. Naturopathic medicine attempts to find the underlying cause of the client's condition rather than focusing solely on their symptoms. Naturopathic doctors (NDs) are preventive medicine specialists and are clinically trained as primary care physicians in natural therapeutics such as physical medicine, clinical nutrition, botanical medicine, homeopathic medicine, environmental medicine, counseling, acupuncture and oriental medicine, and hydrotherapy among others. Their recommendations are based on the individual client, not on the generality of symptoms. This approach has proven successful in treating both chronic and acute conditions.[6]

_____

[6] http://www.scnm.edu/about/naturopathic-medicine

www.ingramcontent.com/pod-product-compliance
Lightning Source LLC
Chambersburg PA
CBHW070817290526
45795CB00002B/738